The Ultimate Coaching Guide

GLAMXY NEO

Table Of Contents

Introduction

Coaching is a collaborative and goal-oriented process that empowers individuals or groups to enhance their personal and professional development. It involves a coach facilitating a client's self-discovery, growth, and performance improvement by providing guidance, support, and accountability.

Purpose of Coaching:

The primary purpose of coaching is to help clients unlock their potential, maximize their performance, and achieve their desired outcomes. Coaching focuses on the present and future, aiming to bridge the gap between where clients are and where they want to be.

Historical Background

Origins of Coaching:

Coaching as a formal discipline emerged in the latter half of the 20th century, drawing influences from various fields such as sports coaching, psychology, management, and leadership training. Key figures like Timothy Gallwey, with his book "The Inner Game of Tennis" (1974), highlighted the mcntal aspcct of performance, laying the groundwork for modern coaching.

Evolution of Coaching:

Coaching has evolved from its initial focus on sports to encompass a wide range of areas, including business, life, career, and executive coaching. The development of coaching methodologies and the establishment of professional bodies, such as the International Coach Federation (ICF) in 1995, have formalized coaching as a respected profession.

 Key Principles of Coaching
Confidentiality: Confidentiality is foundational to the coaching relationship. It ensures that the information shared between the coach and the client remains private, fostering a safe and trusting environment. This principle encourages openness and honesty, which are crucial for effective coaching.

Empathy:
Empathy involves understanding and sharing the feelings and perspectives of the client. By showing empathy, coaches build rapport and create a supportive atmosphere. This helps clients feel valued and understood, which enhances their engagement in the coaching process.

Active Listening:
Active listening goes beyond hearing words; it involves fully concentrating, understanding, and responding to

the client. This skill allows coaches to grasp the client's needs, challenges, and goals, facilitating more meaningful and productive conversations. Accountability: Coaching emphasizes accountability, where clients take responsibility for their actions and progress. Coaches help clients set clear goals, develop action plans, and hold them accountable for their commitments, fostering a sense of ownership and motivation.

Benefits of Coaching

Personal Growth:
Coaching supports individuals in identifying their strengths, values, and aspirations. It helps them overcome limiting beliefs, develop new skills, and enhance their self-awareness, leading to greater personal fulfillment and growth.

Professional Development:
In a professional context, coaching aids in developing leadership skills,

improving performance, and navigating career transitions. It empowers clients to set and achieve career goals, enhance their productivity, and build effective relationships.

Improved Performance: Coaching can lead to significant improvements in performance by helping clients clarify their objectives, stay focused, and implement effective strategies. Whether in sports, business, or personal life, coaching fosters a continuous improvement mindset.

Enhanced Decision-Making: Through coaching, clients develop critical thinking and problem-solving skills. Coaches guide clients in exploring options, evaluating outcomes, and making informed decisions, which enhances their confidence and capability in handling complex situations.

Coaching vs. Other Disciplines

Coaching vs. Therapy:

While both coaching and therapy aim to support individuals' well-being, they differ in focus and approach. Therapy often addresses past issues and emotional healing, while coaching is future-oriented, focusing on goals and actionable steps. Coaches do not diagnose or treat mental health conditions, instead, they help clients move forward from a functional baseline. Coaching vs. Mentoring: Mentoring involves a more experienced individual providing advice and guidance based on their expertise. In contrast, coaching is a partnership where the coach facilitates the client's self-discovery and growth without necessarily being an expert in the client's field. Coaches use questioning and

active listening to help clients find their own solutions.
Coaching vs. Consulting: Consultants provide expert advice and solutions to specific problems, often based on their specialized knowledge.
Coaches, however, help clients develop their own solutions and strategies through a process of inquiry and reflection.
Coaching is more about empowering clients to harness

their potential rather than providing direct answers.

 Conclusion

The introduction to coaching provides a foundation for understanding the core elements and principles of coaching. By focusing on confidentiality, empathy, active listening, and accountability, coaches create a supportive environment that fosters personal and professional growth. The evolution of coaching, its benefits, and its distinction from other disciplines highlight its unique value in helping individuals and organizations achieve their goals.

Types Of Coaching

Coaching comes in various forms, each tailored to specific areas of personal and professional development. Here, we explore some of the most common types of coaching:

1. Executive Coaching

Focus: Executive coaching is designed for leaders, executives, and managers to enhance their leadership skills, strategic thinking, and overall organizational performance. It aims to develop the leadership capacity of individuals within a corporate or organizational context.

Key Areas:

- Leadership Development: Enhancing leadership qualities such as decision-making, vision-setting, and team management.
- Strategic Thinking: Cultivating the ability to think strategically and make long-term plans.
- Performance Management: Improving personal and team performance through effective management techniques.

-         Change Management: Navigating and leading through organizational change and transformation.
Typical Clients:
-         CEOs, executives, senior managers, and high-potential leaders within organizations.
Common Techniques:
-         360-degree feedback assessments, leadership assessments, and personalized development plans.
 2. Life Coaching

Focus:
Life coaching is aimed at individuals seeking personal growth, life balance, and fulfillment. It addresses a broad range of life aspects, helping clients identify and achieve personal goals.
Key Areas:
-       Personal Development: Enhancing self-awareness, confidence, and personal skills.
-       Life Balance: Managing time and energy across various life

domains (e.g., work, family, health).
- Goal Setting: Defining and pursuing personal goals and aspirations.
- Well-being: Improving overall life satisfaction and well-being.
Typical Clients:
- Individuals looking to make positive changes in their personal lives, find balance, or pursue new directions.
Common Techniques:
- Vision boards, journaling, mindfulness

practices, and value assessments.

3. Career Coaching

Focus:

Career coaching helps individuals navigate their professional lives, including career transitions, job searches, and professional development. It aims to align personal strengths and interests with career opportunities.

Key Areas:

- Career Transition: Assisting with career changes,

job searches, and career planning.

- Professional Development: Enhancing skills, performance, and professional growth.
- Resume and Interview Preparation: Crafting resumes, preparing for interviews, and job search strategies.
- Work-Life Integration: Balancing professional and personal responsibilities.

Typical Clients:
- Job seekers, professionals considering a

career change, recent graduates, and individuals aiming for career advancement.

Common Techniques:

- Career assessments, mock interviews, resume workshops, and networking strategies.

4. Performance Coaching

Focus:

Performance coaching is centered on improving an individual's performance in specific areas, whether in sports, business, or other fields. It focuses on setting and achieving high-performance goals.

Key Areas:
- Skill Development: Enhancing specific skills related to the client's performance area.
- Goal Achievement: Setting and achieving challenging performance goals.
- Motivation and Focus: Maintaining motivation and focus to reach peak performance.

- Feedback and Improvement: Providing constructive feedback and identifying areas for continuous improvement.

Typical Clients:

- Athletes, professionals in high-performance roles, and individuals seeking to excel in a specific area.

Common Techniques:

- Performance metrics, regular feedback sessions, visualization techniques, and practice routines.

5. Health and Wellness Coaching
Focus:
Health and wellness coaching supports individuals in achieving optimal health and well-being through lifestyle and behavior changes. It covers physical health, mental well-being, and overall life quality.
Key Areas:
- Nutrition and Exercise: Developing healthy eating habits and fitness routines.
- Stress Management:

Techniques for managing and reducing stress.
- Habit Formation: Establishing and maintaining healthy habits.
- Mental Health: Enhancing mental well-being through mindfulness and other practices.
Typical Clients:
- Individuals seeking to improve their health, manage chronic conditions, or achieve specific wellness goals.
Common Techniques:
- Personalized wellness plans, stress reduction

techniques, mindfulness practices, and accountability structures.

6. Relationship Coaching

Focus: Relationship coaching helps individuals and couples improve their personal and professional relationships. It aims to enhance communication, resolve conflicts, and build stronger, healthier relationships.

Key Areas:
- Communication Skills: Improving listening and

speaking skills to enhance understanding.
-        Conflict Resolution: Techniques for resolving disagreements and conflicts effectively.
-        Relationship Building: Strengthening bonds and building healthy relationships.
-        Personal Boundaries: Establishing and respecting personal boundaries.
Typical Clients:
-        Couples, individuals

looking to improve their relationships, and professionals aiming to enhance workplace relationships.

Common Techniques:
- Communication exercises, role-playing scenarios, and conflict resolution strategies.

7. Financial Coaching

Focus:
Financial coaching assists individuals in managing their finances, creating budgets, and planning for financial goals. It aims to improve

financial literacy and help clients achieve financial stability and success.

Key Areas:

- Budgeting: Creating and maintaining a budget.

- Debt Management: Strategies for reducing and managing debt.

- Savings and Investment: Planning for savings and making informed investment decisions.

- Financial Goals: Setting and achieving short-term and long-term financial goals.

Typical Clients:
- Individuals seeking to improve their financial situation, manage debt, or plan for financial goals.

Common Techniques:
- Financial assessments, budgeting tools, and personalized financial plans.

Conclusion

Understanding the various types of coaching allows both coaches and clients to choose the most appropriate approach for their specific needs and goals. Each type of coaching offers unique benefits and focuses on different aspects of personal and professional development, making coaching a versatile and valuable tool for achieving success and fulfillment in various areas of life.

Coaching Models And Frameworks

Effective coaching often relies on

structured models and frameworks that provide a clear, systematic approach to the coaching process. These models help coaches guide their clients through stages of self-discovery, goal-setting, action planning, and reflection. Here are some of the most widely used coaching models and frameworks:

1. GROW Model

Overview:

The GROW Model is one of the most popular and straightforward coaching frameworks. It stands for Goal, Reality, Options, and Will. This model helps structure coaching sessions and conversations by focusing on four key stages.

Stages:

1. Goal:

- Define what the client wants to achieve.

- Ensure goals are SMART (Specific, Measurable, Achievable, Relevant, Time-bound).

Example Questions:

- What do you want to achieve in this session?
- What is your long-term goal?
- How will you know when you have achieved your goal?

2. Reality:
- Assess the current situation.
- Understand the context and challenges faced by the client.

Example Questions:
- What is happening now?
- What have you tried so far?
- What obstacles are you facing?

3. Options:

- Explore possible strategies and solutions.
- Encourage creative thinking and brainstorming.

Example Questions:
- What options do you have?
- What could you do differently?
- What are the pros and cons of each option?

4. Will:
- Establish commitment to action.
- Develop a clear action plan and set next steps.

Example Questions:

- What will you do next?
- When will you start?
- How will you stay motivated and accountable?

2. CLEAR Model Overview:

The CLEAR Model is a comprehensive framework that emphasizes contracting, active listening, exploration, action planning, and review. It provides a structured approach to coaching conversations and ongoing sessions.

Stages:

1. Contracting:

- Establish the coaching agreement and session goals.

- Clarify expectations, roles, and responsibilities.

Example Questions:

- What do you want to achieve from this session?

- How will we know when we have been successful?

2. Listening:

- Engage in active listening to understand the client's perspective.

- Build rapport and trust.

Example Techniques:

- Reflective listening, summarizing, and acknowledging emotions.

3. Exploring:

- Investigate the client's situation, thoughts, and feelings.

- Identify underlying issues and patterns.

Example Questions:

- What are the main challenges you are facing?

- How do you feel about your current situation?

4. Action:

- Develop actionable steps and strategies.

- Encourage the client to take concrete actions towards their goals.

Example Questions:

- What actions will you take to move forward?

- What resources do you need to implement your plan?

5. Review:

- Reflect on progress and outcomes.

- Adjust the action plan based on feedback and results.

Example Questions:
- What progress have you made since our last session?
- What have you learned from your actions?

3. OSKAR Model

Overview:

The OSKAR Model focuses on solutions and positive outcomes. It stands for Outcome, Scaling, Know-How, Affirm & Action, and Review. This model is particularly useful for solution-focused coaching.

Stages:

1. Outcome:
  - Define the desired outcome of the coaching session or overall goal.

  Example Questions:
  - What do you want to achieve by the end of this session?
  - What does success look like for you?

2. Scaling:
  - Assess the client's current position on a scale relative to their goal.
  - Use scaling questions to measure progress and motivation.

Example
Questions:
- On a scale of 1 to 10, where are you now regarding your goal?
- What would it take to move from a 5 to a 6?
3. Know-How:
- Identify the client's knowledge, skills, and resources.
- Recognize existing strengths and capabilities.
Example
Questions:
- What skills or knowledge do you have that can help you achieve your goal?

- What resources are available to you?

4. Affirm & Action:
- Affirm the client's strengths and successes.
- Develop specific actions to move forward.

Example Questions:
- What steps will you take to achieve your goal?
- How will you leverage your strengths to take these actions?

5. Review:
- Reflect on progress and achievements.

- Adjust the plan as necessary based on outcomes.

Example Questions:
- What progress have you made so far?
- What have you learned from your actions?

4. FUEL Model

Overview:
The FUEL Model provides a structured approach for leadership coaching and performance improvement. It stands for Frame the Conversation, Understand the Current State,

Explore the Desired State, and Lay Out a Success Plan.

Stages:

1. Frame the Conversation:

- Set the context and purpose of the coaching session.

- Establish a positive and collaborative tone.

Example Questions:

- What do we want to focus on today?

- How can we best use our time together?

2. Understand the Current State:

- Assess the client's current

situation and challenges.
- Gather relevant information and insights.
Example Questions:
- What is the current situation?
- What challenges are you facing?
3. Explore the Desired State:
- Define the client's vision for the future.
- Identify goals and desired outcomes.
Example Questions:
- What does success look like for you?

- What are your specific goals?

4. Lay Out a Success Plan:

- Develop a detailed action plan.

- Identify resources, timelines, and support needed.

Example Questions:

- What steps will you take to achieve your goals?

- How will you measure success?

5. SMART Model Overview:

The SMART Model is a goal-setting framework that ensures goals are well-defined and achievable. It stands for Specific, Measurable, Achievable, Relevant, and Time-bound.

Components:

1. Specific:
   - Clearly define the goal with precise details.

   Example:
   - Increase sales by 15% within the next quarter.

2. Measurable:
   - Ensure the goal can be measured and tracked.

   Example:
   - Track sales metrics and compare them to the previous quarter.

3. Achievable:
- Set realistic and attainable goals.
Example:
- Based on current sales trends and resources, a 15% increase is achievable.

4. Relevant:
- Align the goal with broader objectives and values.
Example:
- Increasing sales aligns with the company's growth strategy.

5. Time-bound:
- Set a clear deadline for achieving the goal.
Example:

- Achieve the sales increase by the end of the next quarter.

Conclusion

Coaching models and frameworks provide a structured approach to the coaching process, ensuring that sessions are focused, productive, and goal-oriented. By using models such as GROW, CLEAR, OSKAR, FUEL, and SMART, coaches can effectively guide their clients through stages of self-discovery, goal setting, action planning, and reflection, ultimately helping them achieve their personal and professional objectives.

Essential Coaching Skills

To be an effective coach, it's crucial to develop a range of skills that facilitate growth, learning, and transformation in clients. Here are some of the most important coaching skills:

1. Communication Skills

Questioning:

- Open-Ended Questions: Encourage clients to explore their thoughts and feelings deeply. Examples include, "What are your thoughts on this?" and "How do you feel about this situation?"

- Powerful Questions: Designed to provoke thought and insight, such as "What is the one thing you could do today that would make the biggest difference?" or "What is holding you back from achieving your goal?"

- Clarifying Questions: Ensure understanding and gather more details. For example, "Can you explain what you mean by that?" or "Can you give me an example?"

Active Listening:

- Full Attention: Giving the client your undivided attention and showing interest in what they are saying.

- Reflective Listening:

Paraphrasing and summarizing what the client has said to show understanding and to confirm comprehension. For instance, "So, what you're saying is...?"

- Non-Verbal Cues: Using body language, eye contact, and nodding to show engagement and understanding.

Feedback:

- Constructive Feedback: Providing feedback that is specific, actionable, and focused on

behaviors rather than personal traits. For example, "When you did X, it had Y impact."
- Positive Reinforcement: Recognizing and affirming the client's strengths and successes to build confidence and motivation.
- Balanced Feedback: Combining positive feedback with areas for improvement to provide a comprehensive perspective.
Non-verbal Communication:

- Body Language: Using gestures, facial expressions, and posture to convey attentiveness and empathy.
- Eye Contact: Maintaining appropriate eye contact to show engagement and build rapport.
- Tone of Voice: Modulating your voice to convey interest, concern, or enthusiasm as appropriate.
2. Emotional Intelligence
Self-Awareness:
- Recognizing Emotions: Being aware of your own

emotions and how they affect your thoughts and behavior.
- Reflective Practice: Regularly reflecting on your experiences and feelings to understand your emotional responses better.
Self-Regulation:
- Managing Emotions: Controlling or redirecting disruptive emotions and adapting to changing circumstances.
- Stress Management: Using techniques

such as deep breathing, mindfulness, or exercise to manage stress.

Empathy:

- Understanding Others: Sensing others' emotions, understanding their perspective, and taking an active interest in their concerns.

- Empathetic Listening: Listening with the intention to understand the client's emotional state and perspective fully.

Social Skills:

- Building Rapport:

Establishing a connection with the client based on trust and mutual respect.

- Conflict Resolution: Helping clients navigate and resolve conflicts constructively.

- Influence: Persuading and encouraging clients to take action and make positive changes.

3. Goal Setting and Planning

SMART Goals:

- Specific: Clearly defining the goal. For example, "Increase sales by

10% in the next quarter."

- Measurable: Ensuring the goal can be tracked and measured. For instance, "Track weekly sales reports to monitor progress."

- Achievable: Setting realistic and attainable goals. Example: "Based on past performance, a 10% increase is realistic."

- Relevant: Aligning the goal with broader objectives. Example: "This goal supports the

company's growth strategy."
- Time-bound: Setting a deadline. Example: "Achieve the sales increase by the end of Q2."
Action Planning:
- Breaking Down Goals: Dividing larger goals into smaller, manageable tasks.
- Prioritization: Identifying and focusing on high-priority tasks.
- Timelines: Creating timelines for each task to ensure steady progress.
Motivation and Accountability:

- Inspiring Action: Encouraging clients to take proactive steps toward their goals.
- Tracking Progress: Regularly reviewing progress and adjusting plans as necessary.
- Holding Accountable: Ensuring clients take responsibility for their actions and commitments.

4. Problem-Solving and Decision-Making

Identifying Issues:
- Root Cause Analysis: Helping clients identify the

underlying causes of their problems.
- Brainstorming: Encouraging clients to generate a wide range of potential solutions.
Evaluating Options:
- Pros and Cons Analysis: Weighing the advantages and disadvantages of different options.
- Scenario Planning: Considering various scenarios and their potential outcomes.
Decision-Making:
- Choosing the Best Option:

Assisting clients in selecting the most viable solution.

- Implementation Planning: Developing a plan to put the chosen solution into action.

- Review and Adjust: Evaluating the effectiveness of the decision and making adjustments as necessary.

5. Building Trust and Rapport

Establishing Trust:

- Consistency: Being reliable and consistent in your actions and words.

- Integrity: Acting with honesty and

integrity in all interactions.
- Confidentiality: Ensuring that all client information remains confidential.
Creating a Safe Environment:
- Non-Judgmental Attitude: Providing a safe space for clients to express themselves without fear of judgment.
- Empathy and Understanding: Showing genuine concern and understanding for the client's situation.

Cultural Sensitivity:
- Respect for Diversity: Acknowledging and respecting the client's cultural background and values.
- Cultural Competence: Understanding and appropriately responding to cultural differences.
6. Facilitation Skills
Guiding Discussions:
- Structured Approach: Keeping conversations

focused and productive.

- Inclusiveness: Encouraging all participants to contribute.

Managing Group Dynamics:

- Conflict Management: Addressing and resolving conflicts within a group.

- Encouraging Participation: Ensuring all voices are heard and valued.

Effective Meeting Management:

- Agenda Setting: Preparing and adhering to an agenda.

- Time Management: Ensuring meetings are efficient and productive.

7. Adaptability and Flexibility
Adapting to Client Needs:

- Tailoring Approaches: Modifying coaching methods to suit individual client needs and preferences.

- Responsive Coaching: Being flexible in responding to changing circumstances and client needs.

Learning and Development:

- Continuous Improvement: Seeking feedback and continually improving coaching skills.

- Professional Development: Engaging in ongoing learning and professional development activities.

Conclusion

Mastering these essential coaching skills enables coaches to create meaningful and impactful relationships with their clients. By developing strong communication skills, emotional intelligence, goal-setting capabilities, problem-solving techniques, and the ability to build trust, coaches can effectively guide their clients towards achieving their personal and professional goals. Adaptability and a commitment to continuous improvement are also crucial for staying relevant and effective in the ever-evolving field of coaching.

Coaching Techniques And Tools

Effective coaching involves a variety of techniques and tools designed to help clients achieve their goals, overcome obstacles, and maximize their potential. Below is an expanded overview of essential coaching techniques and tools.

1. Active Listening Technique:

- Full Engagement:

Listen attentively without interrupting.
Focus entirely on what the client is saying.
- Reflecting and Paraphrasing: Repeat back what the client has said in your own words to show understanding and validate their feelings.
- Summarizing: Summarize key points to ensure clarity and understanding.
Tools:
- Listening Exercises: Practicing with scenarios to

improve listening skills.

- Feedback Forms: Using forms to track and reflect on listening effectiveness during sessions.

2. Powerful Questioning Technique:

- Open-Ended Questions: Encourage deeper exploration with questions that cannot be answered with a simple 'yes' or 'no'. Example: "What are your main concerns about this situation?"

- Probing Questions: Delve

deeper into specific areas. Example: "Can you tell me more about that?"
- Hypothetical Questions: Explore possibilities. Example: "What would happen if you tried this approach?"
Tools:
- Question Banks: Collections of effective questions for various scenarios.
- Question Cards: Cards with different types of questions that can be used during sessions to

stimulate discussion.

 3. Goal Setting Technique:

- SMART Goals: Setting goals that are Specific, Measurable, Achievable, Relevant, and Time-bound.

- Backward Planning: Starting with the end goal and planning backward to identify necessary steps.

Tools:

- Goal Setting Worksheets: Templates to help clients define and track their goals.

- Vision Boards: Visual representations of goals and aspirations to keep clients motivated and focused.

4. Action Planning Technique:

- Step-by-Step Planning: Breaking down goals into manageable steps.

- Resource Identification: Identifying the resources and support needed to achieve goals.

- Timeline Creation: Establishing timelines for each

step to ensure progress.
Tools:
- Action Plan Templates: Structured templates to outline steps, resources, and timelines.
- Project Management Software: Tools like Trello or Asana to track progress and keep tasks organized.
5. Feedback and Reflection
Technique:
- Constructive Feedback: Providing specific, actionable feedback focused

on behaviors and outcomes.
- Reflective Practice: Encouraging clients to reflect on their experiences, actions, and outcomes to gain insights.
Tools:
- Feedback Forms: Structured forms to provide and receive feedback.
- Journaling: Encouraging clients to keep a journal to reflect on their thoughts, progress, and learning.
6. Behavioral Coaching
Technique:

- Positive Reinforcement: Reinforcing desirable behaviors to encourage repetition.
- Behavioral Contracting: Establishing agreements on specific behaviors and actions to be taken.
Tools:
- Behavior Charts: Visual charts to track and reinforce positive behaviors.
- Contracts: Written agreements outlining specific commitments and actions.

7. Cognitive Behavioral Techniques (CBT)
Technique:
- Thought Records: Helping clients track and evaluate their thoughts, emotions, and behaviors.
- Reframing: Assisting clients in changing negative thought patterns to more positive ones.
Tools:
- CBT Worksheets: Tools for identifying and challenging negative thoughts.
- Thought Journals: Diaries

for recording and reflecting on thoughts and emotions.

8. Motivational Interviewing Technique:

- Expressing Empathy: Showing understanding and acceptance of the client's perspective.

- Developing Discrepancy: Helping clients see the gap between their current behavior and their goals.

- Rolling with Resistance: Avoiding direct confrontation and instead helping clients find their own solutions.

Tools:

- MI Questionnaires: Structured questions to guide motivational interviews.

- Readiness Rulers: Scales to assess and discuss a client's readiness to change.

9. Visualization and Imagery

Technique:

- Guided Imagery: Leading clients through mental exercises to visualize success and positive outcomes.

- Future Pacing: Helping clients envision their future selves achieving their goals.

Tools:

- Visualization Scripts: Pre-written scripts for guided imagery sessions.

- Vision Boards: Visual tools to represent goals and motivate clients.

10. Strengths-Based Coaching

Technique:

- Identifying Strengths: Helping clients recognize and leverage their strengths.

- Strengths Utilization: Encouraging clients to apply their strengths to overcome challenges and achieve goals.

Tools:

- Strengths Assessments: Tools like Gallup StrengthsFinder to identify individual strengths.

- Strengths Journals: Diaries for clients to record and reflect on the use of their strengths.

11. Mindfulness and Stress Reduction Technique:

- Mindfulness Meditation: Teaching clients techniques to focus on the present moment and reduce stress.
- Breathing Exercises: Helping clients use controlled breathing to manage stress and anxiety.
Tools:
- Mindfulness Apps: Apps like Headspace or Calm for guided mindfulness and meditation.
- Stress Logs: Diaries to track stress levels and identify triggers.

12. Accountability Mechanisms
Technique:
- Regular Check-Ins: Scheduled sessions to review progress and keep clients accountable.
- Accountability Partners: Encouraging clients to pair up with someone who will support and hold them accountable.
Tools:
- Progress Trackers: Tools for tracking and reviewing progress toward goals.
- Accountability Agreements:

Written agreements outlining commitments and responsibilities.
 Conclusion
A diverse set of coaching techniques and tools enhances the effectiveness of coaching by addressing various client needs and preferences. By mastering these techniques and using the appropriate tools, coaches can provide structured, supportive, and impactful guidance that

helps clients achieve their personal and professional goals.

Coaching Process

The coaching process is a structured yet flexible approach that helps clients identify their goals, overcome obstacles, and achieve personal and professional growth. Here is an in-depth look at the stages of the coaching process, including key activities and techniques used in each stage:

1. Establishing the Coaching Relationship

Initial Consultation:

- Purpose: To determine if the coach and client are a good fit and to establish the foundation for the coaching relationship.

- Activities:

- Discussing the client's needs, expectations, and goals.

- Outlining the coaching process and what it entails.

- Addressing any questions or

concerns the client may have.

Setting Boundaries and Expectations:

- Purpose: To ensure both parties are clear on their roles, responsibilities, and the scope of the coaching relationship.

- Activities:
 - Agreeing on confidentiality and ethical guidelines.
 - Defining the frequency and duration of coaching sessions.
 - Establishing the method of communication (in-person, phone,

video conferencing, etc.).
Creating a Coaching Agreement:
- Purpose: To formalize the coaching relationship and outline the terms of engagement.
- Activities:
- Drafting a written agreement that includes session frequency, duration, fees, and cancellation policies.
- Both parties reviewing and signing the agreement.

2. Assessment and Goal Setting
Initial Assessment:
- Purpose: To gain a comprehensive understanding of the client's current situation, strengths, weaknesses, and areas for improvement.
- Activities:
 - Conducting interviews or discussions to gather background information.
 - Using assessment tools (e.g., personality tests, 360-degree feedback) to gather data.

Identifying Goals:
- Purpose: To define clear, specific, and achievable goals that the client wants to work towards.
- Activities:
 - Engaging in goal-setting conversations using frameworks like SMART (Specific, Measurable, Achievable, Relevant, Time-bound).
 - Prioritizing goals based on their importance and impact.
Creating an Action Plan:

- Purpose: To outline the steps the client needs to take to achieve their goals.
- Activities:
  - Breaking down goals into smaller, manageable tasks.
  - Establishing timelines and milestones for each task.
  - Identifying resources and support needed to complete tasks.

3. Coaching Sessions

Regular Coaching Sessions:
- Purpose: To provide ongoing support, guidance, and accountability

as the client works towards their goals.
- Activities:
    - Reviewing progress since the last session.
    - Discussing challenges and obstacles.
    - Brainstorming solutions and strategies.
Techniques Used in Sessions:
- Active Listening: Fully engaging with the client's words and emotions to understand their perspective.
- Powerful Questioning: Asking open-

ended questions to stimulate reflection and insight.
- Example: "What's the most significant challenge you're facing right now?"
- Feedback and Reflection: Providing constructive feedback and encouraging the client to reflect on their experiences.
- Visualization: Guiding the client through exercises to visualize their success and plan their actions.
- Mindfulness and Stress Reduction:

Teaching techniques like mindfulness meditation and breathing exercises to manage stress.

4. Monitoring and Adjusting the Plan Tracking Progress:
- Purpose: To ensure the client is on track to achieve their goals and to make necessary adjustments.
- Activities:
  - Using progress tracking tools like action plan templates or project management software.

- Regularly reviewing and discussing progress in coaching sessions.

Adjusting Goals and Plans:

- Purpose: To adapt to new insights, challenges, or changes in the client's situation.

- Activities:

 - Revisiting and revising goals as needed.

 - Adjusting action steps and timelines based on progress and feedback.

5. Overcoming Obstacles

Identifying Barriers:
- Purpose: To recognize and understand the obstacles that are hindering the client's progress.
- Activities:
  - Discussing and analyzing the client's challenges.
  - Identifying patterns or recurring issues.
Developing Strategies:
- Purpose: To create effective solutions for overcoming obstacles.
- Activities:

- Brainstorming possible solutions and strategies.
- Evaluating the pros and cons of each option.
- Implementing the chosen strategies and monitoring their effectiveness.

6. Building Skills and Capabilities

Skill Development:

- Purpose: To enhance the client's skills and capabilities to achieve their goals.
- Activities:
- Identifying skills that need improvement.

-       Providing training, resources, or exercises to develop these skills.

Capability Building:

-       Purpose: To strengthen the client's overall ability to perform effectively in various situations.

- Activities:

-       Encouraging continuous learning and professional development.

- Supporting the client in taking on new challenges and responsibilities.

7. Review and Evaluation
Regular Reviews:
- Purpose: To assess the overall progress and effectiveness of the coaching process.
- Activities:
  - Conducting periodic reviews to evaluate progress toward goals.
  - Soliciting feedback from the client on the coaching process.
Final Evaluation:
- Purpose: To reflect on the outcomes of the coaching engagement and plan for future steps.

- Activities:
  - Reviewing the achievements and progress made during the coaching engagement.
  - Discussing next steps and future goals.
  - Formalizing the end of the coaching relationship or planning for ongoing support if needed.

Conclusion

The coaching process is a dynamic and iterative journey that requires active engagement, continuous assessment, and adaptation. By following a structured approach, coaches can provide meaningful support that empowers clients to achieve their goals, overcome challenges, and realize their full potential. Each stage of the process is essential in building a strong coaching relationship, facilitating growth, and ensuring sustained success.

Ethical Considerations

Ethical considerations are fundamental to establishing trust, credibility, and professionalism in coaching. Coaches must adhere to ethical standards to ensure that their practices are aligned with the best interests of their clients and uphold the integrity of the coaching profession. Below are key ethical considerations in coaching:

1. Confidentiality

Importance:

- Maintaining confidentiality is crucial for building trust and ensuring that clients feel safe to share personal and sensitive information.

Practices:

- Clear Agreements: Establish clear confidentiality agreements at the beginning of the coaching relationship. Discuss what information will be kept

confidential and under what circumstances, if any, information may need to be disclosed (e.g., legal requirements).
- Secure Records: Keep all client records, notes, and communications secure and confidential. Use encrypted storage systems for digital records and ensure physical documents are locked away.
- Boundary Setting: Avoid discussing client information with third parties

unless explicit consent is given by the client.

2. Informed Consent
Importance:
- Clients must be fully informed about the coaching process, methods, potential risks, and benefits to make knowledgeable decisions about their participation.
Practices:
- Comprehensive Agreements: Provide detailed coaching agreements that outline the scope of coaching, session frequency,

duration, fees, confidentiality policies, and the coach's qualifications.
- Transparency: Be transparent about the coaching methods and techniques used. Explain the rationale behind each approach and ensure the client understands and agrees to them.
- Right to Withdraw: Inform clients of their right to withdraw from coaching at any time without penalty.
3. Professional Boundaries

Importance:
- Maintaining professional boundaries ensures that the coaching relationship remains appropriate, respectful, and focused on the client's goals.
Practices:
- Role Clarity: Clearly define the role of the coach and distinguish it from other roles such as friend, therapist, or consultant.
- Avoid Dual Relationships: Avoid entering into dual

relationships with clients that could impair objectivity, professionalism, or client welfare. Examples include personal, business, or social relationships.

- Appropriate Conduct: Maintain appropriate physical and emotional boundaries. Refrain from engaging in any form of relationship with a client that could be considered inappropriate or exploitative.

4. Competence
Importance:

- Coaches must possess the necessary skills, knowledge, and experience to provide effective coaching services.

Practices:

- Continual Learning: Engage in ongoing professional development and training to stay current with coaching practices and methodologies.

- Supervision and Peer Support: Participate in supervision or peer coaching groups to gain feedback and

support for continuous improvement.
- Scope of Practice: Recognize and respect the limits of your competence. Refer clients to other professionals (e.g., therapists, counselors) when issues arise that are beyond the scope of coaching.
5. Conflict of Interest
Importance:
- Managing conflicts of interest is essential to maintain impartiality and

prioritize the client's best interests.
Practices:
- Disclosure: Disclose any potential conflicts of interest at the outset of the coaching relationship. This includes any personal, financial, or business relationships that may influence the coaching process.
- Client Interests First: Always prioritize the client's interests above your own or any third party's interests.

- Independent Decision-Making: Avoid situations where your judgment may be compromised. Ensure that your coaching decisions are made independently and solely for the benefit of the client.

6. Respect for Diversity and Inclusion

Importance:

- Respecting diversity and promoting inclusion ensures that coaching is accessible, equitable, and respectful of all individuals.

Practices:

- Cultural Competence: Develop an understanding of different cultural backgrounds, values, and perspectives. Engage in cultural competence training and education.

- Non-Discriminatory Practices: Ensure that coaching practices are free from discrimination based on race, ethnicity, gender, sexual orientation,

age, disability, religion, or any other characteristic.
- Inclusive Environment: Create an environment where all clients feel respected, valued, and understood. Tailor coaching approaches to meet the diverse needs of clients.
7. Integrity and Honesty
Importance:
- Integrity and honesty are foundational to building trust and credibility in the

coaching relationship.
Practices:
- Truthfulness: Be honest and truthful in all communications with clients. Provide accurate information about your qualifications, experience, and the coaching process.
- Ethical Marketing: Ensure that all marketing and promotional materials accurately represent your services and do not make false or misleading claims.

- Honest Feedback: Provide honest and constructive feedback to clients, even when it may be challenging to hear. Focus on supporting the client's growth and development.

8. Accountability
Importance:
- Accountability ensures that coaches are responsible for their actions and decisions, maintaining high professional standards.
Practices:

- Professional Memberships: Join and adhere to the ethical guidelines of professional coaching organizations (e.g., International Coaching Federation, European Mentoring and Coaching Council).
- Regular Review: Regularly review and reflect on your coaching practice to ensure adherence to ethical standards.
- Feedback Mechanisms: Implement mechanisms for

clients to provide feedback on the coaching experience. Use this feedback to improve and refine your practice.

9. Termination of Coaching Relationship

Importance:

- Ethical termination ensures that the coaching relationship ends in a manner that is respectful and beneficial for the client.

Practices:

- Clear Process: Establish and communicate a clear process for

the termination of
the coaching
relationship at the
outset.
- Mutual
Agreement:
Whenever
possible,
terminate the
coaching
relationship by
mutual agreement.
Ensure that the
client feels
supported during
the transition.
- Referral: If
coaching is no
longer beneficial
or appropriate,
refer the client to
other
professionals or
resources that may

better meet their needs.

 Conclusion

Ethical considerations are integral to the practice of coaching. By adhering to ethical guidelines and principles, coaches can build trust, foster a positive coaching environment, and provide effective and responsible support to their clients. Ensuring confidentiality, informed consent, professional boundaries, competence, conflict of interest management, respect for diversity, integrity, accountability, and ethical termination are all crucial components of ethical coaching practice.

Continuous Improvement

Continuous improvement is essential for coaches to stay effective, relevant, and professional. It involves a commitment to ongoing learning, self-assessment, and adaptation to new coaching practices and client needs. Here is an expanded overview of strategies and practices for continuous improvement in coaching:

1. Professional Development

Ongoing Education:

- Certifications and Courses: Pursue advanced certifications and specialized courses offered by recognized coaching organizations.

Examples include ICF-accredited programs, NLP certification, or courses in positive psychology.
- Workshops and Seminars: Attend workshops, seminars, and conferences to learn about the latest trends, tools, and techniques in coaching.
Reading and Research:
- Books and Journals: Regularly read books, peer-reviewed journals, and articles related to coaching,

psychology, leadership, and personal development.

- Research Studies: Stay informed about new research and evidence-based practices in coaching and related fields.

Webinars and Online Learning:

- Webinars: Participate in webinars hosted by coaching organizations, universities, or industry experts.

- Online Courses: Enroll in online courses through platforms like

Coursera, Udemy, or edX to gain new skills and knowledge.

2. Supervision and Mentoring

Coaching Supervision:

- Regular Supervision Sessions: Engage in regular supervision with an experienced coach supervisor to reflect on your coaching practice, discuss challenges, and receive constructive feedback.

- Case Studies: Present and discuss case studies from your

coaching practice to gain new perspectives and insights.
Mentoring:
- Finding a Mentor: Seek out a mentor who is an experienced coach to guide you, provide feedback, and share their knowledge and experiences.
- Mentoring Others: Act as a mentor to less experienced coaches. This not only helps them but also reinforces your own knowledge and skills.

3. Peer Coaching and Support Groups

Peer Coaching:

- Reciprocal Coaching: Partner with another coach for reciprocal coaching sessions. This allows you to experience coaching from the client's perspective and receive feedback on your own practice.

- Peer Feedback: Provide and receive feedback from peers on coaching techniques, approaches, and

session effectiveness.
Support Groups:
- Coaching Circles: Join or form coaching circles or support groups where coaches can share experiences, discuss challenges, and learn from each other.
- Discussion Forums: Participate in online discussion forums and communities for coaches to exchange ideas and support.
4. Self-Reflection and Self-Assessment

Reflective Practice:

- Journaling: Maintain a reflective journal to record your thoughts, experiences, and insights after each coaching session. Reflect on what went well, what could be improved, and what you learned.

- Self-Questioning: Regularly ask yourself questions such as, "What did I do well in this session?", "What could I have done differently?", and "What will I try next time?"

Self-Assessment Tools:
- Competency Frameworks: Use coaching competency frameworks (e.g., ICF Core Competencies) to assess your skills and identify areas for development.
- Feedback Surveys: Develop and use feedback surveys for clients to provide anonymous feedback on your coaching practice.

5. Feedback and Evaluation

Client Feedback:
- Regular Feedback: Solicit

regular feedback from clients about their coaching experience, the effectiveness of sessions, and areas for improvement.

- Exit Surveys: Use exit surveys at the end of the coaching engagement to gather comprehensive feedback on your performance and the overall coaching process.

360-Degree Feedback:

- Holistic Feedback: Implement 360-degree feedback processes to receive input from clients, peers, supervisors, and other stakeholders.

6. Adapting and Innovating

Staying Current:

- Industry Trends: Stay informed about current trends, new techniques, and innovations in coaching. Follow industry leaders, read coaching blogs, and subscribe to coaching newsletters.

- Technology Integration: Incorporate new technologies and

tools into your coaching practice. This could include virtual coaching platforms, AI-powered coaching apps, or digital assessment tools.
Experimentation and Innovation:
- New Techniques: Experiment with new coaching techniques and approaches to find what works best for different clients and situations.
- Creative Approaches: Be open to creative and unconventional methods that can

enhance the coaching experience and outcomes.

7. Quality Assurance Standards and Best Practices:

- Adherence to Standards: Ensure that your coaching practice adheres to the standards and best practices set by professional coaching organizations (e.g., ICF, EMCC).

- Ethical Practice: Regularly review and update your ethical guidelines and ensure they are aligned with current standards.

Quality Control Measures:

- Session Reviews: Regularly review and evaluate your coaching sessions, either independently or with a supervisor, to ensure quality and consistency.

- Client Outcomes: Track and measure client outcomes to assess the effectiveness of your coaching interventions and adjust your approach as necessary.

8. Networking and Community Engagement

Professional Networks:

- Join Coaching Associations: Become a member of professional coaching associations to access resources, training, and networking opportunities.
- Networking Events: Attend industry events, meet-ups, and networking sessions to connect with other coaches and professionals.

Community Involvement:

- Pro Bono Coaching: Offer

pro bono coaching to non-profits, community organizations, or individuals who cannot afford coaching. This not only contributes to your community but also provides diverse coaching experiences.

- Volunteer Work: Engage in volunteer work related to coaching, such as speaking at events, writing articles, or mentoring aspiring coaches.

 Conclusion

Continuous improvement is an ongoing

commitment that enables coaches to enhance their skills, stay current with industry trends, and provide the highest quality service to their clients. By engaging in professional development, seeking supervision and mentoring, participating in peer coaching and support groups, practicing self-reflection and self-assessment, gathering feedback, adapting and innovating, maintaining quality assurance, and networking, coaches can ensure they remain effective, relevant, and impactful in their coaching practice.

Case Studies And Success Stories

Case studies and success stories are powerful tools for illustrating the impact of coaching and demonstrating how coaching techniques can be applied to achieve tangible results.

They provide real-world examples that can inspire and inform both coaches and clients. Below, we delve into the importance of case studies and success stories, and provide detailed examples in various coaching contexts.

Importance of Case Studies and Success Stories

Real-World Applications:

- Case studies demonstrate how coaching theories and techniques are applied in real-world scenarios,

bridging the gap between theory and practice.
Evidence of Effectiveness:
- Success stories provide evidence of the effectiveness of coaching, showcasing measurable outcomes and client achievements.
Learning Opportunities:
- Analyzing case studies allows coaches to learn from different approaches, challenges, and solutions, enhancing their own practice.

Inspiration and Motivation:
- Success stories can motivate and inspire clients by showing that others have successfully navigated similar challenges and achieved their goals.

Detailed Case Studies and Success Stories

1. Executive Coaching

Case Study: Leadership Development

Client Profile:
- Senior executive at a mid-sized technology company facing

challenges in team management and strategic planning.
Coaching Objectives:
- Improve leadership skills, enhance team communication, and develop a strategic vision for the company.
Process:
- Initial Assessment: Conducted 360-degree feedback and a leadership skills assessment to identify strengths and areas for improvement.
- Goal Setting: Established

specific, measurable goals for leadership development, including improving delegation skills and fostering a collaborative team environment.

- Coaching Sessions: Focused on developing emotional intelligence, effective communication strategies, and strategic thinking. Used role-playing exercises to practice new behaviors.

- Action Plan: Created a detailed

action plan with steps to implement strategic initiatives and improve team dynamics.
Outcome:
- The executive reported significant improvements in team engagement and productivity. The company saw a 15% increase in project completion rates and a noticeable enhancement in overall employee morale.
2. Career Coaching
Case Study: Career Transition
Client Profile:

- Mid-career professional in the finance industry seeking a transition to a more fulfilling career in environmental sustainability.

Coaching Objectives:

- Identify transferable skills, explore career options in sustainability, and develop a plan for transitioning to a new field.

Process:

- Career Assessment: Conducted a comprehensive career assessment to identify the client's strengths, interests, and values.

- Exploration: Guided the client through exploring various roles in the sustainability sector, including informational interviews with professionals in the field.

- Skill Development: Identified key skills needed for the new career path and created a development plan, including relevant certifications and networking opportunities.

- Job Search Strategy: Developed a targeted job search strategy, including resume and cover letter revisions, LinkedIn profile optimization, and interview preparation.

Outcome:

- The client successfully transitioned to a role as a sustainability analyst within six months. They reported increased job satisfaction and a sense of purpose in their new career.

3. Life Coaching

Case Study: Work-Life Balance

Client Profile:

- Busy professionals and parents struggling to balance work responsibilities with family life and personal well-being.

Coaching Objectives:

- Achieve a healthier work-life balance, reduce stress, and improve overall well-being.

Process:

- Initial Assessment: Used a work-life balance assessment tool to identify areas of

imbalance and sources of stress.
- Goal Setting: Established goals for reducing work hours, increasing family time, and incorporating self-care practices.
- Time Management: Implemented time management techniques, such as prioritization, delegation, and time-blocking.
- Self-Care Plan: Developed a self-care plan that included regular exercise, meditation, and hobbies.

-     Boundaries: Worked on setting clear boundaries between work and personal life, including setting limits on after-hours work communication.
Outcome:
-     The client achieved a more balanced lifestyle, reporting reduced stress levels and improved relationships with family members. Their productivity at work also increased, leading to a promotion within the year.
4.   Performance Coaching

Case Study: Enhancing Sales Performance

Client Profile:

- Sales manager at a retail company looking to improve the performance of their sales team.

Coaching Objectives:

- Increase sales team performance, enhance motivation, and develop effective sales strategies.

Process:

- Performance Assessment: Conducted an assessment of the sales team's performance metrics and

identified key areas for improvement.
- Training and Development: Provided targeted training on advanced sales techniques, customer relationship management, and negotiation skills.
- Motivation Strategies: Implemented motivational strategies, including setting achievable targets, providing regular feedback, and creating incentive programs.

- Coaching
Sessions:
Conducted regular
coaching sessions
with the sales
manager to
develop leadership
skills and effective
team management
practices.
Outcome:
- The sales team's
performance
improved
significantly, with
a 20% increase in
monthly sales and
higher customer
satisfaction
ratings. The sales
manager reported
enhanced team
morale and
motivation.

5. Wellness Coaching

Case Study: Weight Loss and Healthy Living

Client Profile:

- Individual seeking to lose weight and adopt a healthier lifestyle.

Coaching Objectives:

- Achieve sustainable weight loss, develop healthy eating habits, and incorporate regular physical activity into daily routine.

Process:

- Initial Assessment: Conducted a

health and lifestyle assessment to understand the client's current habits, challenges, and goals.
- Goal Setting: Established realistic and achievable weight loss and wellness goals.
- Nutrition Plan: Developed a personalized nutrition plan with the help of a dietitian, focusing on balanced meals and mindful eating practices.
- Exercise Routine: Created a tailored exercise routine that included both

cardiovascular and strength training activities.

- Behavioral Change Techniques: Used techniques such as habit tracking, positive reinforcement, and visualization to support behavior change.

Outcome:

- The client lost 25 pounds over six months and reported increased energy levels and improved self-esteem. They successfully maintained their new healthy habits and continued to work towards additional wellness goals.

Conclusion

Case studies and success stories are valuable tools for demonstrating the impact and effectiveness of coaching. They provide concrete examples of how coaching can lead to significant personal and professional growth, inspire others, and offer practical insights into the coaching process. By examining these real-world applications, coaches can refine their techniques, while clients can gain confidence in the potential benefits of coaching.

Resources

A variety of resources are available to support the continuous growth and development of coaches. These resources can help coaches stay informed about industry trends, enhance their skills, and maintain high standards of practice. Below is an expanded overview of valuable resources for coaches.

1. Professional Organizations and Associations
International Coaching Federation (ICF):
- Overview: The ICF is a leading global organization dedicated to advancing the coaching profession.
- Resources:
 - Credentialing Programs: Provides certification and

credentialing for coaches.

- ICF Core Competencies: Offers a set of core competencies to guide coaching practices.

- ICF Research Portal: Access to research articles and studies related to coaching.

- Networking Opportunities: Local chapters, conferences, and events for networking and professional development.

European Mentoring and Coaching Council (EMCC):

- Overview: The EMCC promotes best practices and standards in mentoring and coaching across Europe and beyond.
- Resources:
  - Accreditation: Offers individual and organizational accreditation.
  - Competence Framework: Provides a comprehensive framework for coaching competencies.
  - Events and Webinars: Hosts regular events and webinars on

various coaching topics.

Association for Coaching (AC):

- Overview: The AC is an international association dedicated to promoting excellence and ethics in coaching.

- Resources:

  - Accreditation Programs: Offers accreditation for coaches and coaching training programs.

  - Member Resources: Access to a library of articles, case studies, and tools.

-     Professional Development: Workshops, webinars, and conferences for ongoing learning.

2.   Educational Programs and Training

University Programs:

-     Graduate Certificates and Degrees: Many universities offer graduate certificates, master's degrees, and doctoral programs in coaching, psychology, and leadership.

-     Example: Harvard Extension

School offers a Graduate Certificate in Organizational Behavior focusing on coaching.

Specialized Training Institutes:

- Coaching Training Programs: Numerous institutes provide specialized training in coaching methodologies and techniques.

- Example: The Coaches Training Institute (CTI) offers the Co-Active Coach training program.

Online Learning Platforms:

\- Coursera, Udemy, edX: These platforms offer a range of courses in coaching, leadership, and personal development.

\- Example: Coursera offers a course on "Coaching Skills for Managers" by the University of California, Davis.

3. Books and Publications

Foundational Books:

\- "Co-Active Coaching" by Karen Kimsey-

House, Henry Kimsey-House, Phil Sandahl, and Laura Whitworth:
- A comprehensive guide to the co-active coaching model.
- "The Coaching Habit" by Michael Bungay Stanier:
- Practical advice on how to develop effective coaching habits.
- "Quiet Leadership" by David Rock:
- Focuses on how to bring out the best in people through coaching.
Journals and Magazines:

- International Journal of Evidence-Based Coaching and Mentoring:
 - Publishes research articles and case studies related to coaching.
- Coaching World (ICF):
 - A digital magazine offering insights, trends, and tips for coaches.
- Choice Magazine:
 - Focuses on professional coaching and offers articles on coaching practices,

tools, and techniques.

4. Tools and Assessments

Personality and Behavioral Assessments:

- Myers-Briggs Type Indicator (MBTI):
  - Assesses personality types and helps clients understand their preferences.
- DiSC Assessment:
  - Measures behavioral styles and helps improve communication and teamwork.
- StrengthsFinder (CliftonStrengths):

- Identifies clients' strengths and helps leverage them for personal and professional growth.
Coaching Platforms:
-
CoachAccountable:
- A comprehensive coaching management platform for tracking client progress, scheduling sessions, and managing administrative tasks.
- BetterUp:

- Provides a digital coaching platform with tools for goal setting, tracking, and feedback.

Action Planning Tools:

- Trello and Asana:
 - Project management tools that help coaches and clients organize tasks, set deadlines, and track progress.

5. Supervision and Peer Support

Coaching Supervision

Services:

- Supervisors: Engage with qualified coaching supervisors who

provide oversight, feedback, and support.
    - Example: Coaching Supervision Academy offers supervision training and services.
Peer Coaching Networks:
    - Peer Groups: Join peer coaching groups or networks where coaches can practice skills, share experiences, and receive feedback.
    - Example: The ICF offers local chapter meetings

and peer coaching opportunities.
Mentoring Programs:
- Mentorship Opportunities: Seek out or become a mentor through professional coaching organizations.
 - Example: The Association for Coaching offers a mentoring program for its members.
 6. Research and Insights
Research Databases:
- Google Scholar:
 - Access to a wide range of scholarly

articles and research papers on coaching and related fields.
- ResearchGate:
 - A network for researchers to share and access research publications.
Industry Reports:
- ICF Global Coaching Study:
 - Provides comprehensive data and insights on the coaching industry.
- Market Research Reports:
 - Reports from firms like IBISWorld and MarketResearch.com offer industry

trends and market analysis.

7. Networking and Community Engagement

Professional Conferences:

- ICF Converge:

  - An annual global coaching conference offering networking, learning, and development opportunities.

- World Business and Executive Coach Summit (WBECS):

  - A virtual summit featuring leading experts in the coaching industry.

Online Communities:

- LinkedIn Groups:
  - Join LinkedIn groups focused on coaching to connect with peers and engage in discussions.
  - Example: International Coaching Federation Group on LinkedIn.

Local Meetups:
- Meetup.com:
  - Find and join local coaching meetups to network with other coaches and professionals.

Conclusion

A wealth of resources is available to support the continuous growth and development of coaches. By leveraging professional organizations, educational programs, books, tools, supervision, research, and networking opportunities, coaches can enhance their skills, stay informed about industry trends, and provide high-quality services to their clients. Continuous engagement with these resources ensures that coaches remain effective, ethical, and impactful in their practice.

Conclusion

Coaching is a dynamic and evolving profession that requires a deep commitment to personal and professional growth. The ultimate coaching guide has covered various aspects essential to becoming a successful and impactful coach. By integrating these components, coaches can enhance their effectiveness, foster meaningful client relationships, and achieve sustainable outcomes.

1. Understanding Coaching

Coaching is a powerful process that facilitates personal and professional growth. It involves helping clients set and achieve their goals, overcome obstacles, and develop new skills. By understanding the essence of coaching, its principles, and its benefits, coaches can create a solid foundation for their practice.

2. Types of Coaching

Coaching comes in many forms, each tailored to specific contexts and client needs. From executive coaching to wellness coaching, understanding the different types enables coaches to specialize and offer targeted support. This specialization allows for more precise and effective interventions, leading to better client outcomes.

3. Coaching Models and Frameworks Utilizing established coaching models and frameworks provides structure and consistency to the coaching process. Models such as GROW, SMART, and CLEAR help coaches guide their clients through a systematic

approach to goal setting and achievement. Familiarity with these frameworks allows coaches to adapt their techniques to best suit each client's unique situation.

4. Essential Coaching Skills

Effective coaching relies on a set of core skills, including active listening, powerful questioning, and empathy. These skills enable coaches to build rapport, understand client needs, and facilitate transformative conversations. Continuous practice and refinement of these skills are crucial for maintaining high standards of coaching practice.

5. Coaching Techniques and Tools

A wide array of techniques and tools can enhance the coaching process. From personality assessments to visualization exercises, these tools help clients gain insights, track progress, and stay motivated. Coaches should be proficient in selecting and applying these techniques to maximize their impact.

6. The Coaching Process

A structured coaching process ensures that clients move systematically towards their goals. This process typically includes stages such as assessment, goal setting, action planning, and review. By following a clear process, coaches can provide consistent and reliable support to their clients.

7. Ethical Considerations

Adhering to ethical standards is paramount in coaching. Coaches must maintain confidentiality, set clear boundaries, and practice with integrity and honesty. Ethical coaching fosters trust, respect, and professionalism, which are essential for effective client relationships.

8. Continuous Improvement

Coaching is a field that requires lifelong learning and adaptation. Continuous improvement involves engaging in professional development, seeking supervision, and staying informed about industry trends. By committing to continuous improvement, coaches can enhance their skills, stay relevant, and provide the best possible service to their clients.

9. Case Studies and Success Stories

Sharing case studies and success stories highlights the transformative power of coaching. These real-world examples demonstrate how coaching techniques can lead to significant personal and professional growth. They provide inspiration and practical insights for both coaches and clients.

10. Resources

A wealth of resources is available to support coaches in their journey. Professional organizations, educational programs, books, tools, and networking opportunities all contribute to a coach's development. Leveraging these resources ensures that coaches remain informed, skilled, and effective in their practice.

Integrating It All: The Ultimate Coaching Journey

The ultimate coaching guide offers a comprehensive roadmap for coaches at any stage of their career. Whether you are a novice coach just starting out or an experienced professional looking to refine your practice, the principles and strategies outlined in this guide will help you achieve excellence in coaching.

Building a Strong Foundation:
- Begin with a thorough

understanding of the core principles and ethics of coaching. This foundational knowledge will guide all your interactions and decisions.

Specializing and Adapting:

- Identify your niche and specialize in areas that align with your strengths and interests.

Continuously adapt your approach to meet the evolving needs of your clients.

Commitment to Growth:

-      Engage in continuous professional development, seek feedback, and embrace new learning opportunities. This commitment to growth will keep your coaching practice vibrant and effective.

Ethics and Integrity:

- Always uphold the highest standards of ethics and integrity. Trust and respect are the cornerstones of effective coaching relationships.

Leveraging Resources:
- Utilize the vast array of available resources to enhance your skills and knowledge. Professional organizations, educational programs, and networking opportunities are invaluable assets in your coaching journey.
Celebrating Success:
- Celebrate your successes and those of your clients. Recognize the progress made and use these

achievements as motivation to continue striving for excellence.

 Final Thoughts Coaching is more than a profession; it is a calling to facilitate growth, change, and empowerment in others. By integrating the insights and strategies from the ultimate coaching guide, you can create a meaningful and impactful coaching practice that makes a difference in the lives of your clients.

Stay committed to your journey of continuous improvement, embrace the challenges, and celebrate the successes. The path of a coach is one of constant learning and transformation, both for you and those you coach. With dedication, passion, and the right resources, you can become an exceptional coach who inspires and empowers others to reach their fullest potential.

9 798327 728547